I0408479

# Homemade Deodorant
## 30 Best Natural Homemade Deodorant And Body Spray Recipes To Keep You Dry And Smelling Fresh All Day Long!

# Table of content

## Introduction

Another day is here, and you have to get up and go.

You have no time to get in and shower, and you can only hope your hair is going to cooperate with you. You try to eat breakfast as you slip on your clothes for the day, and you know that getting that morning latte is going to be a squeeze with how today is going.

But there's one thing you simply can't overlook.

No matter how rushed you are in the morning, it is essential you take the time to come outside clean and fresh... something that is much easier said than done with your tight schedule.

So what do you do?

There's no time to shower and you know you haven't done laundry as recently as you would have liked, so you have to go with the only option available... the quick fix.

What better way to get you out the door and on your way than with a bit of all natural body spray? The deodorizing power is going to leave you feeling clean and refreshed, and you can feel confident knowing you are all natural and healthy.

So with these recipes on hand, you have everything you need to get your day started on the right track. Try one, try them all, and get out there and show the world what you are made of.

You know you smell good, so strut your stuff.

# Chapter 1 – Fast and Easy Recipes

## *Morning Sunshine*

*What you will need:*

*10 drops cinnamon*

*8 drops chocolate aromatherapy oil*

*8 drops vanilla oil*

*15 drops clary sage oil*

*¼ cup distilled water*

*½ teaspoon apple cider vinegar*

*1/3 cup witch hazel*

*½ cup aloe vera juice*

*1 teaspoon baking soda*

*1 teaspoon lemon juice*

*Directions:*

Combine all ingredients in a spray bottle.

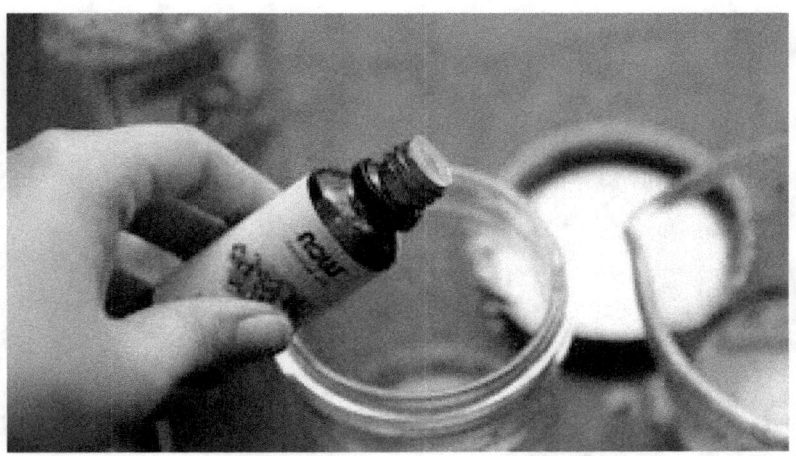

If you want to make more at a time, you can always add more distilled water to fill up the remainder of the jar.

Add in as many of the essential oils as you like, until you are perfectly happy with the scent. I like the amounts I listed for the recipes, but if you want more of one or less of another, feel free to make it happen!

When you are ready to use, shake the bottle well before you begin, and spray on your underarms. Let dry and get dressed as usual.

For use as a body spray, simply spray where desired for a long lasting fresh scent!

## The Quick Fix

*10 drops spearmint*

*8 drops peppermint*

*8 drops grapefruit*

*15 drops clary sage oil*

*¼ cup distilled water*

*½ teaspoon apple cider vinegar*

*1/3 cup witch hazel*

*½ cup aloe vera juice*

*1 teaspoon baking soda*

*1 teaspoon lemon juice*

*Directions:*

Combine all ingredients in a spray bottle.


If you want to make more at a time, you can always add more distilled water to fill up the remainder of the jar.


Add in as many of the essential oils as you like, until you are perfectly happy with the scent. I like the amounts I listed for the recipes, but if you want more of one or less of another, feel free to make it happen!

When you are ready to use, shake the bottle well before you begin, and spray on your underarms. Let dry and get dressed as usual.

For use as a body spray, simply spray where desired for a long lasting fresh scent!

## The Hot Mess

*10 drops sandalwood*

*10 drops rose*

*8 drops jasmine*

*15 drops clary sage oil*

*¼ cup distilled water*

*½ teaspoon apple cider vinegar*

*1/3 cup witch hazel*

*½ cup aloe vera juice*

*1 teaspoon baking soda*

*1 teaspoon lemon juice*

*Directions:*

Combine all ingredients in a spray bottle.

If you want to make more at a time, you can always add more distilled water to fill up the remainder of the jar.

Add in as many of the essential oils as you like, until you are perfectly happy with the scent. I like the amounts I listed for the recipes, but if you want more of one or less of another, feel free to make it happen!

When you are ready to use, shake the bottle well before you begin, and spray on your underarms. Let dry and get dressed as usual.

For use as a body spray, simply spray where desired for a long lasting fresh scent!


## *The Good Day*

*10 drops clean linen aromatherapy oil*

*8 drops lavender*

*8 drops lilac*

*15 drops clary sage oil*

*¼ cup distilled water*

*½ teaspoon apple cider vinegar*

*1/3 cup witch hazel*

*½ cup aloe vera juice*

*1 teaspoon baking soda*

*1 teaspoon lemon juice*

*Directions:*

Combine all ingredients in a spray bottle.

If you want to make more at a time, you can always add more distilled water to fill up the remainder of the jar.

Add in as many of the essential oils as you like, until you are perfectly happy with the scent. I like the amounts I listed for the recipes, but if you want more of one or less of another, feel free to make it happen!

When you are ready to use, shake the bottle well before you begin, and spray on your underarms. Let dry and get dressed as usual.

For use as a body spray, simply spray where desired for a long lasting fresh scent!

## Starting Right Spray

*8 drops peppermint*

*8 drops orange*

*8 drops vanilla essential oil*

*15 drops clary sage oil*

*¼ cup distilled water*

*½ teaspoon apple cider vinegar*

*1/3 cup witch hazel*

*½ cup aloe vera juice*

*1 teaspoon baking soda*

*1 teaspoon lemon juice*

*Directions:*

Combine all ingredients in a spray bottle.

If you want to make more at a time, you can always add more distilled water to fill up the remainder of the jar.

Add in as many of the essential oils as you like, until you are perfectly happy with the scent. I like the amounts I listed for the recipes, but if you want more of one or less of another, feel free to make it happen!

When you are ready to use, shake the bottle well before you begin, and spray on your underarms. Let dry and get dressed as usual.

For use as a body spray, simply spray where desired for a long lasting fresh scent!

## Chapter 2 – Sizzlin' and Sparklin'

### *Faith, Trust, and Dust*

*10 drops goldenseal*

*8 drops grapefruit*

*8 drops cinnamon*

*15 drops clary sage oil*

*¼ cup distilled water*

*½ teaspoon apple cider vinegar*

*1/3 cup witch hazel*

*½ cup aloe vera juice*

*1 teaspoon baking soda*

*1 teaspoon lemon juice*

*Directions:*

Combine all ingredients in a spray bottle.

If you want to make more at a time, you can always add more distilled water to fill up the remainder of the jar.

Add in as many of the essential oils as you like, until you are perfectly happy with the scent. I like the amounts I listed for the recipes, but if you want more of one or less of another, feel free to make it happen!

When you are ready to use, shake the bottle well before you begin, and spray on your underarms. Let dry and get dressed as usual.

For use as a body spray, simply spray where desired for a long lasting fresh scent!

## *Princess's Secret*

*10 drops hibiscus*

*8 drops rose*

*8 drops lavender*

*15 drops clary sage oil*

*¼ cup distilled water*

*½ teaspoon apple cider vinegar*

*1/3 cup witch hazel*

*½ cup aloe vera juice*

*1 teaspoon baking soda*

*1 teaspoon lemon juice*

*Directions:*

Combine all ingredients in a spray bottle.

If you want to make more at a time, you can always add more distilled water to fill up the remainder of the jar.

Add in as many of the essential oils as you like, until you are perfectly happy with the scent. I like the amounts I listed for the recipes, but if you want more of one or less of another, feel free to make it happen!

When you are ready to use, shake the bottle well before you begin, and spray on your underarms. Let dry and get dressed as usual.

For use as a body spray, simply spray where desired for a long lasting fresh scent!

## Always Amazing

*10 drops apple aromatherapy oil*

*10 drops caramel aromatherapy oil*

*15 drops clary sage oil*

*¼ cup distilled water*

*½ teaspoon apple cider vinegar*

*1/3 cup witch hazel*

*½ cup aloe vera juice*

*1 teaspoon baking soda*

*1 teaspoon lemon juice*

*Directions:*

Combine all ingredients in a spray bottle.

If you want to make more at a time, you can always add more distilled water to fill up the remainder of the jar.

Add in as many of the essential oils as you like, until you are perfectly happy with the scent. I like the amounts I listed for the recipes, but if you want more of one or less of another, feel free to make it happen!

When you are ready to use, shake the bottle well before you begin, and spray on your underarms. Let dry and get dressed as usual.

For use as a body spray, simply spray where desired for a long lasting fresh scent!

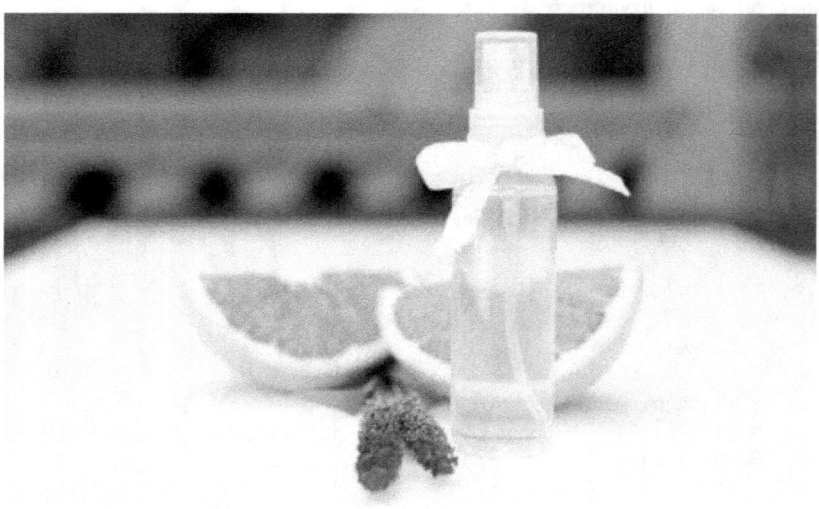

## Catch Me if You Can

*8 drops lavender*

*8 drops saffron*

*8 drops rose*

*15 drops clary sage oil*

*¼ cup distilled water*

*½ teaspoon apple cider vinegar*

*1/3 cup witch hazel*

*½ cup aloe vera juice*

*1 teaspoon baking soda*

*1 teaspoon lemon juice*

*Directions:*

Combine all ingredients in a spray bottle.

If you want to make more at a time, you can always add more distilled water to fill up the remainder of the jar.

Add in as many of the essential oils as you like, until you are perfectly happy with the scent. I like the amounts I listed for the recipes, but if you want more of one or less of another, feel free to make it happen!

When you are ready to use, shake the bottle well before you begin, and spray on your underarms. Let dry and get dressed as usual.

For use as a body spray, simply spray where desired for a long lasting fresh scent!

## *Sunshine and Kisses*

*8 drops bergamot*

*10 drops cardamom*

*15 drops clary sage oil*

*¼ cup distilled water*

*½ teaspoon apple cider vinegar*

*1/3 cup witch hazel*

*½ cup aloe vera juice*

*1 teaspoon baking soda*

*1 teaspoon lemon juice*

*Directions:*

Combine all ingredients in a spray bottle.

If you want to make more at a time, you can always add more distilled water to fill up the remainder of the jar.

Add in as many of the essential oils as you like, until you are perfectly happy with the scent. I like the amounts I listed for the recipes, but if you want more of one or less of another, feel free to make it happen!

When you are ready to use, shake the bottle well before you begin, and spray on your underarms. Let dry and get dressed as usual.

For use as a body spray, simply spray where desired for a long lasting fresh scent!

## Chapter 3 – No Worries Stress Response Recipes

## *Promotion Power*

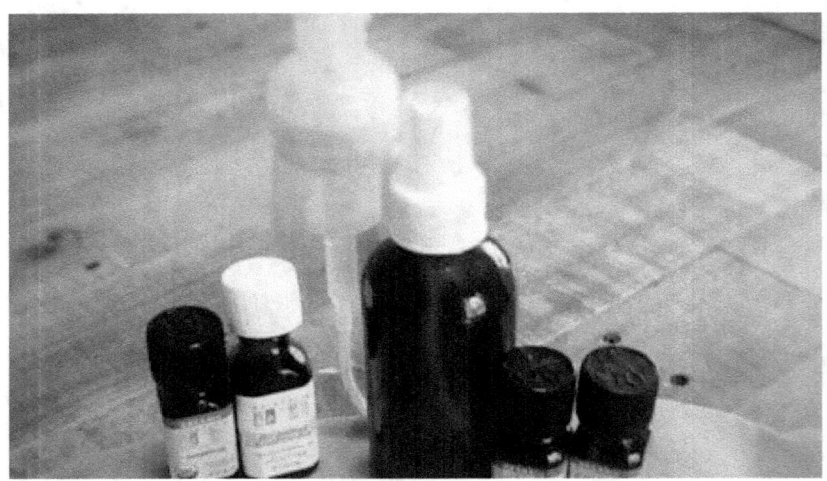

*10 drops ylang ylang*

*8 drops rosewood*

*10 drops cedar*

*15 drops clary sage oil*

*¼ cup distilled water*

*½ teaspoon apple cider vinegar*

*1/3 cup witch hazel*

*½ cup aloe vera juice*

*1 teaspoon baking soda*

*1 teaspoon lemon juice*

*Directions:*

Combine all ingredients in a spray bottle.

If you want to make more at a time, you can always add more distilled water to fill up the remainder of the jar.

Add in as many of the essential oils as you like, until you are perfectly happy with the scent. I like the amounts I listed for the recipes, but if you want more of one or less of another, feel free to make it happen!

When you are ready to use, shake the bottle well before you begin, and spray on your underarms. Let dry and get dressed as usual.

For use as a body spray, simply spray where desired for a long lasting fresh scent!

## Cool and Collected

*10 drops tea tree oil*

*10 drops grapefruit oil*

*15 drops clary sage oil*

*¼ cup distilled water*

*½ teaspoon apple cider vinegar*

*1/3 cup witch hazel*

*½ cup aloe vera juice*

*1 teaspoon baking soda*

*1 teaspoon lemon juice*

*Directions:*

Combine all ingredients in a spray bottle.

If you want to make more at a time, you can always add more distilled water to fill up the remainder of the jar.

Add in as many of the essential oils as you like, until you are perfectly happy with the scent. I like the amounts I listed for the recipes, but if you want more of one or less of another, feel free to make it happen!

When you are ready to use, shake the bottle well before you begin, and spray on your underarms. Let dry and get dressed as usual.

For use as a body spray, simply spray where desired for a long lasting fresh scent!

## Date Night

*10 drops frankincense*

*10 drops myrrh*

*10 drops goldenseal*

*15 drops clary sage oil*

*¼ cup distilled water*

½ teaspoon apple cider vinegar

1/3 cup witch hazel

½ cup aloe vera juice

1 teaspoon baking soda

1 teaspoon lemon juice


*Directions:*

Combine all ingredients in a spray bottle.

If you want to make more at a time, you can always add more distilled water to fill up the remainder of the jar.

Add in as many of the essential oils as you like, until you are perfectly happy with the scent. I like the amounts I listed for the recipes, but if you want more of one or less of another, feel free to make it happen!

When you are ready to use, shake the bottle well before you begin, and spray on your underarms. Let dry and get dressed as usual.

For use as a body spray, simply spray where desired for a long lasting fresh scent!


## The Secret Agent

10 drops white musk aromatherapy oil

10 drops sandalwood

10 drops vanilla essential oil

15 drops clary sage oil

¼ cup distilled water

½ teaspoon apple cider vinegar

1/3 cup witch hazel

½ cup aloe vera juice

1 teaspoon baking soda

1 teaspoon lemon juice


*Directions:*

Combine all ingredients in a spray bottle.

If you want to make more at a time, you can always add more distilled water to fill up the remainder of the jar.

Add in as many of the essential oils as you like, until you are perfectly happy with the scent. I like the amounts I listed for the recipes, but if you want more of one or less of another, feel free to make it happen!

When you are ready to use, shake the bottle well before you begin, and spray on your underarms. Let dry and get dressed as usual.

For use as a body spray, simply spray where desired for a long lasting fresh scent!


## The Cool Cat

10 drops pine

10 drops winter green

10 drops peppermint

*15 drops clary sage oil*

*¼ cup distilled water*

*½ teaspoon apple cider vinegar*

*1/3 cup witch hazel*

*½ cup aloe vera juice*

*1 teaspoon baking soda*

*1 teaspoon lemon juice*

*Directions:*

Combine all ingredients in a spray bottle.

If you want to make more at a time, you can always add more distilled water to fill up the remainder of the jar.

Add in as many of the essential oils as you like, until you are perfectly happy with the scent. I like the amounts I listed for the recipes, but if you want more of one or less of another, feel free to make it happen!

When you are ready to use, shake the bottle well before you begin, and spray on your underarms. Let dry and get dressed as usual.

For use as a body spray, simply spray where desired for a long lasting fresh scent!

## Chapter 4 – Fresh and Fit Recipes

### *Fitness Fun*

*10 drops tea tree oil*

*10 drops geranium*

*15 drops clary sage oil*

*¼ cup distilled water*

*½ teaspoon apple cider vinegar*

*1/3 cup witch hazel*

*½ cup aloe vera juice*

*1 teaspoon baking soda*

*1 teaspoon lemon juice*

*Directions:*

Combine all ingredients in a spray bottle.

If you want to make more at a time, you can always add more distilled water to fill up the remainder of the jar.

Add in as many of the essential oils as you like, until you are perfectly happy with the scent. I like the amounts I listed for the recipes, but if you want more of one or less of another, feel free to make it happen!

When you are ready to use, shake the bottle well before you begin, and spray on your underarms. Let dry and get dressed as usual.

For use as a body spray, simply spray where desired for a long lasting fresh scent!

## Fantastic Four

10 drops peppermint

10 drops spearmint

10 drops cinnamon

10 drops vanilla oil

15 drops clary sage oil

¼ cup distilled water

½ teaspoon apple cider vinegar

1/3 cup witch hazel

½ cup aloe vera juice

1 teaspoon baking soda

1 teaspoon lemon juice

Directions:

Combine all ingredients in a spray bottle.

If you want to make more at a time, you can always add more distilled water to fill up the remainder of the jar.

Add in as many of the essential oils as you like, until you are perfectly happy with the scent. I like the amounts I listed for the recipes, but if you want more of one or less of another, feel free to make it happen!

When you are ready to use, shake the bottle well before you begin, and spray on your underarms. Let dry and get dressed as usual.

For use as a body spray, simply spray where desired for a long lasting fresh scent!

## *Fresh as a Daisy*

*10 drops spearmint*

*10 drops rose*

*10 drops lavender*

*15 drops clary sage oil*

*¼ cup distilled water*

*½ teaspoon apple cider vinegar*

*1/3 cup witch hazel*

*½ cup aloe vera juice*

*1 teaspoon baking soda*

*1 teaspoon lemon juice*

*Directions·*

Combine all ingredients in a spray bottle.

If you want to make more at a time, you can always add more distilled water to fill up the remainder of the jar.

Add in as many of the essential oils as you like, until you are perfectly happy with the scent. I like the amounts I listed for the recipes, but if you want more of one or less of another, feel free to make it happen!

When you are ready to use, shake the bottle well before you begin, and spray on your underarms. Let dry and get dressed as usual.

For use as a body spray, simply spray where desired for a long lasting fresh scent!

## *Run Run Rose*

*10 drops rose*

*10 drops rose wood*

*10 drops vanilla oil*

*15 drops clary sage oil*

*¼ cup distilled water*

*½ teaspoon apple cider vinegar*

*1/3 cup witch hazel*

*½ cup aloe vera juice*

*1 teaspoon baking soda*

*1 teaspoon lemon juice*

*Directions:*

Combine all ingredients in a spray bottle.

If you want to make more at a time, you can always add more distilled water to fill up the remainder of the jar.

Add in as many of the essential oils as you like, until you are perfectly happy with the scent. I like the amounts I listed for the recipes, but if you want more of one or less of another, feel free to make it happen!

When you are ready to use, shake the bottle well before you begin, and spray on your underarms. Let dry and get dressed as usual.

For use as a body spray, simply spray where desired for a long lasting fresh scent!

## Fit and Fabulous

*10 drops cinnamon*

*10 drops rose*

*15 drops clary sage oil*

*¼ cup distilled water*

*½ teaspoon apple cider vinegar*

*1/3 cup witch hazel*

*½ cup aloe vera juice*

*1 teaspoon baking soda*

*1 teaspoon lemon juice*

*Directions:*

Combine all ingredients in a spray bottle.

If you want to make more at a time, you can always add more distilled water to fill up the remainder of the jar.

Add in as many of the essential oils as you like, until you are perfectly happy with the scent. I like the amounts I listed for the recipes, but if you want more of one or less of another, feel free to make it happen!

When you are ready to use, shake the bottle well before you begin, and spray on your underarms. Let dry and get dressed as usual.

For use as a body spray, simply spray where desired for a long lasting fresh scent!

## Chapter 5 – Fun and Fancy Free Recipes

### *A Day at the Beach*

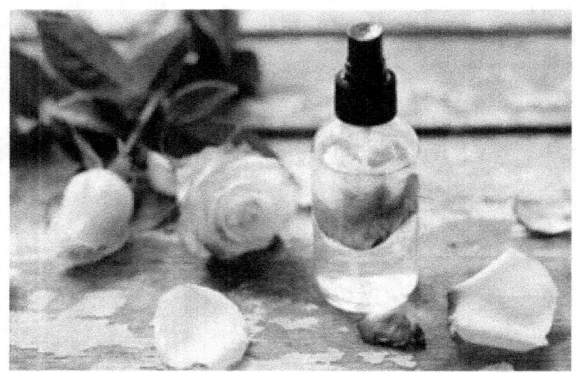

*10 drops grapefruit oil*

*10 drops lemon oil*

*10 drops orange oil*

*15 drops clary sage oil*

*¼ cup distilled water*

*½ teaspoon apple cider vinegar*

*1/3 cup witch hazel*

½ cup aloe vera juice

1 teaspoon baking soda

1 teaspoon lemon juice


*Directions:*

Combine all ingredients in a spray bottle.

If you want to make more at a time, you can always add more distilled water to fill up the remainder of the jar.

Add in as many of the essential oils as you like, until you are perfectly happy with the scent. I like the amounts I listed for the recipes, but if you want more of one or less of another, feel free to make it happen!

When you are ready to use, shake the bottle well before you begin, and spray on your underarms. Let dry and get dressed as usual.

For use as a body spray, simply spray where desired for a long lasting fresh scent!


## When Life Gives You Lemons

10 drops lemon

10 drops lemongrass

5 drops orange

15 drops clary sage oil

¼ cup distilled water

½ teaspoon apple cider vinegar

1/3 cup witch hazel

½ cup aloe vera juice

1 teaspoon baking soda

1 teaspoon lemon juice


*Directions:*

Combine all ingredients in a spray bottle.

If you want to make more at a time, you can always add more distilled water to fill up the remainder of the jar.

Add in as many of the essential oils as you like, until you are perfectly happy with the scent. I like the amounts I listed for the recipes, but if you want more of one or less of another, feel free to make it happen!

When you are ready to use, shake the bottle well before you begin, and spray on your underarms. Let dry and get dressed as usual.

For use as a body spray, simply spray where desired for a long lasting fresh scent!


## On My Tab

10 drops jasmine

5 drops lemongrass

15 drops clary sage oil

¼ cup distilled water

½ teaspoon apple cider vinegar

*1/3 cup witch hazel*

*½ cup aloe vera juice*

*1 teaspoon baking soda*

*1 teaspoon lemon juice*

*Directions:*

Combine all ingredients in a spray bottle.

If you want to make more at a time, you can always add more distilled water to fill up the remainder of the jar.

Add in as many of the essential oils as you like, until you are perfectly happy with the scent. I like the amounts I listed for the recipes, but if you want more of one or less of another, feel free to make it happen!

When you are ready to use, shake the bottle well before you begin, and spray on your underarms. Let dry and get dressed as usual.

For use as a body spray, simply spray where desired for a long lasting fresh scent!

## Night Life

*10 drops white musk aromatherapy oil*

*3 drops tea tree oil*

*15 drops clary sage oil*

*¼ cup distilled water*

*½ teaspoon apple cider vinegar*

1/3 cup witch hazel

½ cup aloe vera juice

1 teaspoon baking soda

1 teaspoon lemon juice

*Directions:*

Combine all ingredients in a spray bottle.

If you want to make more at a time, you can always add more distilled water to fill up the remainder of the jar.

Add in as many of the essential oils as you like, until you are perfectly happy with the scent. I like the amounts I listed for the recipes, but if you want more of one or less of another, feel free to make it happen!

When you are ready to use, shake the bottle well before you begin, and spray on your underarms. Let dry and get dressed as usual.

For use as a body spray, simply spray where desired for a long lasting fresh scent!

## Woke Up Like This

10 drops bubblegum aromatherapy oil

5 drops peppermint

15 drops clary sage oil

¼ cup distilled water

½ teaspoon apple cider vinegar

*1/3 cup witch hazel*

*½ cup aloe vera juice*

*1 teaspoon baking soda*

*1 teaspoon lemon juice*

*Directions:*

Combine all ingredients in a spray bottle.

If you want to make more at a time, you can always add more distilled water to fill up the remainder of the jar.

Add in as many of the essential oils as you like, until you are perfectly happy with the scent. I like the amounts I listed for the recipes, but if you want more of one or less of another, feel free to make it happen!

When you are ready to use, shake the bottle well before you begin, and spray on your underarms. Let dry and get dressed as usual.

For use as a body spray, simply spray where desired for a long lasting fresh scent!

## Chapter 6 – The Best of the Rest

### *Moonlight Fantasy*

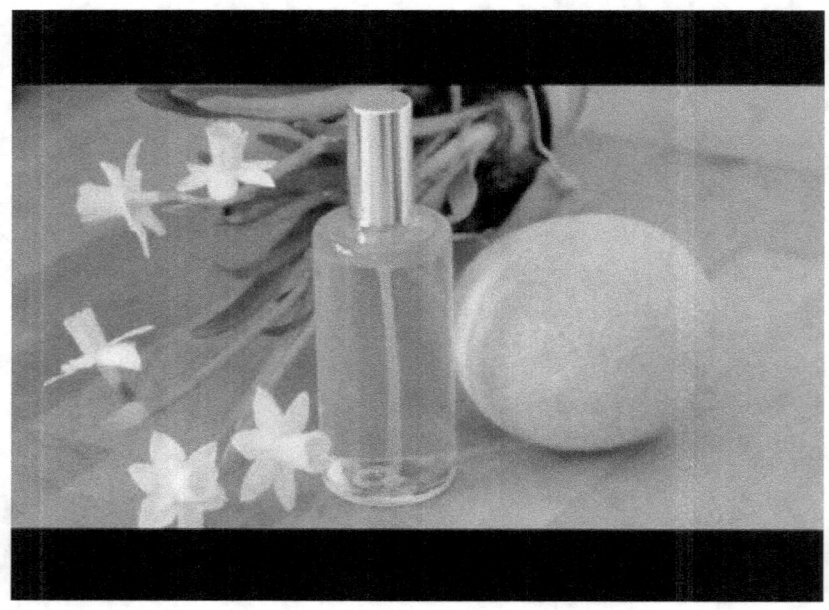

h t t p s : / / w w w . g o o g l e . c o m / s e a r c h ?
q=homemade+body+spray&espv=2&biw=1366&bih=667&source=lnms&tbm=isch&sa=X&ved=0ahUKEwiUr5irxszOAh-
VQwGMKHVjPDfoQ_AUIBygC#imgrc=_

*10 drops frankincense*

*5 drops myrrh*

*15 drops clary sage oil*

¼ cup distilled water

½ teaspoon apple cider vinegar

1/3 cup witch hazel

½ cup aloe vera juice

1 teaspoon baking soda

1 teaspoon lemon juice

Directions:

Combine all ingredients in a spray bottle.

If you want to make more at a time, you can always add more distilled water to fill up the remainder of the jar.

Add in as many of the essential oils as you like, until you are perfectly happy with the scent. I like the amounts I listed for the recipes, but if you want more of one or less of another, feel free to make it happen!

When you are ready to use, shake the bottle well before you begin, and spray on your underarms. Let dry and get dressed as usual.

For use as a body spray, simply spray where desired for a long lasting fresh scent!

## Hush Little Baby

10 drops baby powder aromatherapy oil

5 drops lavender

15 drops clary sage oil

¼ cup distilled water

½ teaspoon apple cider vinegar

1/3 cup witch hazel

½ cup aloe vera juice

1 teaspoon baking soda

1 teaspoon lemon juice

*Directions:*

Combine all ingredients in a spray bottle.

If you want to make more at a time, you can always add more distilled water to fill up the remainder of the jar.

Add in as many of the essential oils as you like, until you are perfectly happy with the scent. I like the amounts I listed for the recipes, but if you want more of one or less of another, feel free to make it happen!

When you are ready to use, shake the bottle well before you begin, and spray on your underarms. Let dry and get dressed as usual.

For use as a body spray, simply spray where desired for a long lasting fresh scent!

## All in a Look

5 drops marjoram

5 drops sandalwood

15 drops clary sage oil

*¼ cup distilled water*

*½ teaspoon apple cider vinegar*

*1/3 cup witch hazel*

*½ cup aloe vera juice*

*1 teaspoon baking soda*

*1 teaspoon lemon juice*

*Directions:*

Combine all ingredients in a spray bottle.

If you want to make more at a time, you can always add more distilled water to fill up the remainder of the jar.

Add in as many of the essential oils as you like, until you are perfectly happy with the scent. I like the amounts I listed for the recipes, but if you want more of one or less of another, feel free to make it happen!

When you are ready to use, shake the bottle well before you begin, and spray on your underarms. Let dry and get dressed as usual.

For use as a body spray, simply spray where desired for a long lasting fresh scent!

**That's What He Said**

*5 drops white musk aromatherapy oil*

*8 drops cedar*

*15 drops clary sage oil*

*¼ cup distilled water*

*½ teaspoon apple cider vinegar*

*1/3 cup witch hazel*

*½ cup aloe vera juice*

*1 teaspoon baking soda*

*1 teaspoon lemon juice*

*Directions:*

Combine all ingredients in a spray bottle.

If you want to make more at a time, you can always add more distilled water to fill up the remainder of the jar.

Add in as many of the essential oils as you like, until you are perfectly happy with the scent. I like the amounts I listed for the recipes, but if you want more of one or less of another, feel free to make it happen!

When you are ready to use, shake the bottle well before you begin, and spray on your underarms. Let dry and get dressed as usual.

For use as a body spray, simply spray where desired for a long lasting fresh scent!

## Hip Hip Happiness

*5 drops patchouli*

*5 drops pine*

*15 drops clary sage oil*

*¼ cup distilled water*

*½ teaspoon apple cider vinegar*

*1/3 cup witch hazel*

*½ cup aloe vera juice*

*1 teaspoon baking soda*

*1 teaspoon lemon juice*

*Directions:*

Combine all ingredients in a spray bottle.

If you want to make more at a time, you can always add more distilled water to fill up the remainder of the jar.

Add in as many of the essential oils as you like, until you are perfectly happy with the scent. I like the amounts I listed for the recipes, but if you want more of one or less of another, feel free to make it happen!

When you are ready to use, shake the bottle well before you begin, and spray on your underarms. Let dry and get dressed as usual.

For use as a body spray, simply spray where desired for a long lasting fresh scent!

## Conclusion

There you have it, everything you need to know to make your own deodorant and body spray, and to make it as unique as you are!

Now you don't need to worry about all of those adverse effects you read about in everyday deodorants, and you can go through your day with confidence, knowing you smell great and feel fantastic.

So if you are ready to take on the world with a fresh new perspective, you have come to the right place...

Now get out there and work your magic.

# FREE Bonus Reminder

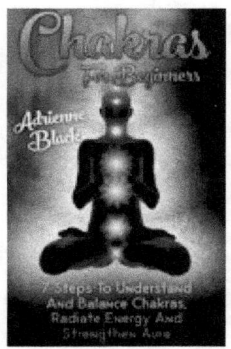

If you have not grabbed it yet, please go ahead and download your special bonus E book *"Chakras for Beginners. 7 Steps To Understand And Balance Chakras, Radiate Energy, And Strengthen Aura"*.

## Simply Click the Button Below

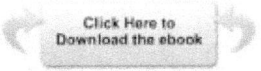

## OR Go to This Page

### http://lifehacksworld.com/free

## BONUS #2: More Free & Discounted Books & Products

### Do you want to receive more Free/Discounted Books or Products?

We have a mailing list where we send out our new Books or Products when they go free or with a discount on Amazon. Click on the link below to sign up for Free & Discount Book & Product Promotions.

### => Sign Up for Free & Discount Book & Product Promotions <=

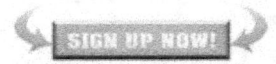

OR Go to this URL

http://zbit.ly/1WBb1Ek

www.ingramcontent.com/pod-product-compliance
Lightning Source LLC
Chambersburg PA
CBHW071300280526
45788CB00004B/1785